ULTIMATE LOW CARB DIET BOOK FOR SENIORS

EPIPHANY HUB PRINTS

ULTIMATE LOW CARB DIET BOOK FOR SENIORS

COPYRIGHT © [2023] BY [EPIPHANY HUB PRINTS]

TABLE OF CONTENTS

INTRODUCTION

The importance of a carefully planned diet cannot be emphasized in the quest for peak health and energy in old age. With years of experience as a senior nutrition specialist, I'm excited to share with you the life-changing potential of the Ultimate Low Carb Diet.

This dietary approach supports the special nutritional demands of older adults and promotes a lifestyle that enables people to age gracefully and vibrantly. It is not just a fad. It is a well-thought-out, scientifically supported approach.

Seniors frequently have unique metabolic, muscle-maintenance, and general health issues. The Ultimate Low Carb Diet for Seniors shows up as a nutritional lighthouse, providing a way forward that not only tackles these issues but also improves quality of life.

This diet helps to maintain stable blood sugar levels, which is important for controlling energy levels and lowering the risk of chronic illnesses like diabetes. It does this by limiting the amount of carbohydrates consumed.

The Ultimate Low Carb Diet's emphasis on maintaining lean muscle mass is one of its main advantages for senior citizens. Maintaining muscle becomes more and more important as we age for strength, movement, and independence. This diet's deliberate cutbacks on carbohydrates urge the body to burn fat reserves instead of energy, protecting valuable muscle mass. This promotes general physical function as well as weight management.

Moreover, the Senior Ultimate Low Carb Diet is a formidable foe in the fight against inflammation, a common adversary that can exacerbate a host of age-related illnesses. The inclusion of nutrient-dense, low-carbohydrate foods that are high in antioxidants and anti-inflammatory qualities makes this diet an effective tool for supporting cardiovascular health, cognitive function, and joint health.

Starting the Ultimate Low Carb Diet for Seniors is more than simply a decision about what to eat; it's a commitment to giving your body the best fuel possible.

Come along on this dietary adventure designed to greet the golden years with vigor, resiliency, and a delicious selection of nutritious options. Your health should never settle for anything less than the best nutrition available, and together, we can open the doors to a more vibrant, healthy senior years.

THANK YOU VERY MUCH FOR TAKING YOUR TIME TO READ THIS BOOK. I FOUND JOY SHARING MY THOUGHTS WITH YOU. HAVING ENJOYED **"ULTIMATE LOW CARB DIET BOOK FOR SENIORS"**, I WOULD DROP OUR EMAIL AS A MEANS OF REACHING OUT.

MEANWHILE I SENT OUT READING LIST OF MY FAVORITE BOOKS FROM MYSELF AND OTHER AUTHORS ON A WIDE RANGE OF SUBJECTS.

epiphanyhubprints@gmail.com

I ALWAYS HAVE A GIFT FOR EVERYONE THAT REACHED OUT!

IN OUR BOOK SHELF WE'VE ALREADY CREATED

"THE ULTIMATE LOW CARB DIET RECIPES COOKBOOK FOR BEGINNERS"

HERE IS THE LINK …PLEASE CLICK!

"EMPOWER YOUR GOLDEN YEARS WITH LOW CARB CHEERS!"

CHAPTER 1:

LOW CARB NUTRITION FOR SENIORS:

As we become older, our nutritional needs alter, and what we eat can have a significant effect on our general health. One nutritional approach that has grown in favor is the low-carb diet, which is especially beneficial for senior citizens. We will discuss the fundamentals of low-carb nutrition for seniors in this session, along with its benefits and an explanation of the principles of carbohydrates in relation to the optimal low-carb diet.

Advantages of a Low Carb Diet for Seniors

Weight management: Seniors can more successfully maintain their weight with a low-carb diet. Cutting less on carbs promotes the body to burn fat reserves for energy, which could lead to weight loss or maintenance.

Blood Sugar Control: For seniors with diabetes or at risk for the condition, a low-carb diet can help control blood sugar levels. Cutting back on carbohydrates reduces blood glucose spikes and crashes, which aids with condition management.

Heart Health: Reducing carbs is one way to improve heart health. Low-carb diets often result in lower triglycerides, higher HDL (good) cholesterol, and fewer heart disease risk factors.

Mental Clarity: Seniors who eat a low-carb diet report being more cognitively efficient and having improved mental clarity. Stable blood sugar levels and decreased inflammation can support enhanced brain function.

Reduced Inflammation: Inflammation is linked to several age-related diseases. Low-carb diets have the potential to reduce inflammatory markers, which could benefit senior citizens by reducing their risk of chronic illness.

Control Your Appetite: Overindulging in food or picking unhealthy snacks is a common issue among senior citizens. Low-carb diets can help with appetite control since they lower cravings and stabilize blood sugar.

Knowing the Fundamentals of Carbohydrates

Along with proteins and fats, carbohydrates are one of the three main macronutrients. They provide the body with energy and can take many different forms, including fiber, sugars, and carbs. Seniors should be aware of the following details:

Simple vs. Complex carbs: Simple carbs are more readily absorbed and raise blood sugar levels than complex carbs. They can be found in processed snacks and sugary meals. Vegetables, legumes, and whole grains all contain complex carbs. They digest more slowly and provide you with energy that lasts longer.

Fiber: Fiber is a type of carbohydrate that the body does not fully digest. It is necessary for promoting fullness, controlling blood sugar, and preserving digestive health.

Net carbohydrates: The focus of a low-carb diet is generally on "net carbs," which are calculated by subtracting the grams of fiber from the total number of carbohydrates. This provides a more accurate representation of how carbohydrates affect blood sugar levels.

"SENIOR WELLNESS: WHERE LOW CARBS TAKE THE LEAD."

CHAPTER 2:

THE SENIOR'S GUIDE TO LOW CARB MEAL PLANNING

Our nutritional needs change as we age, so choosing wisely what to eat is essential to living a long and healthy life. A low-carb diet can be quite beneficial for many seniors, especially those who are seeking to regulate their weight or blood sugar levels. We'll examine "The Ultimate low carb Diet for Seniors," which was created specifically with the unique needs and challenges that older people face in mind. In our archive we've already created "The Ultimate Low Carb Diet Recipes Cookbook for Beginners"

Setting Your Daily Carbohydrate Goals:

Establishing your daily carbohydrate objectives is one of the most important steps in beginning a low-carb diet. Individual differences exist in the optimal consumption of carbohydrates due to variables such as age, degree of physical activity, and medical problems. Seniors who want to set individualized carbohydrate goals that support their health goals should speak with a qualified dietician or their healthcare physician. Reducing processed carbohydrates and sugars while including complete, nutrient-dense foods like vegetables, lean meats, and healthy fats is frequently the focus of these objectives.

Creating Balanced Low Carb Meals:

A balanced low-carb diet is the cornerstone of any successful senior diet plan. To achieve this balance, consider including a variety of nutrient-rich foods in your meals. To maintain muscle mass, choose for lean protein sources such as fish, poultry, and tofu.

Add non-starchy vegetables like leafy greens, broccoli, and cauliflower to get your recommended daily allowance of vitamins and fiber. Nutritious fats found in foods like avocados, almonds, and olive oil can help with satiety and overall health. Furthermore, bear in mind that meals with a low glycemic index, like berries, may enable you to satisfy your sweet tooth without increasing blood sugar levels.

Tips for Portion Control:

Portion control is crucial for seniors who wish to efficiently control their consumption of carbohydrates. Because their demands for calories are often lower than in their younger years, portion control is even more crucial for older adults.

Use smaller plates, measure portions, and pay attention to your body's hunger and fullness cues. If you eat in moderation, you can have delicious low-carb meals without going crazy.

"The Ultimate low carb Diet for Seniors" offers seniors who want to begin a personalized low-carb diet incisive analysis and helpful advice. Seniors who prepare balanced low-carb meals, exercise portion control, and set personalized carbohydrate targets can enhance their nutritional well-being and reap the many benefits of a low-carb diet.

To create a personalized plan that considers your medical history and health goals, consult a dietitian or other healthcare professional.

"GOLDEN YEARS, GOLDEN CARBS – THE ULTIMATE SENIOR DIET."

CHAPTER 3:

ESSENTIAL NUTRIENTS FOR SENIOR HEALTH ON AN ULTIMATE LOW CARB DIET

Seniors who aim to maintain a healthy lifestyle must make important dietary decisions in order to preserve their physical and emotional well-being. In the framework of the optimal low-carb diet for seniors, three essential nutrients stand out: fiber, protein, and vitamins and minerals. These nutrients are critical for preserving general health, gut health, and muscular strength in seniors following a low-carb diet.

1. Protein and Muscle Maintenance:

Protein is essential for older people since it is the building block of muscle. Strength, mobility, and overall functionality all depend on maintaining muscle mass. For a low-carb diet, lean meats, fish, poultry, tofu, and dairy products are great sources of protein. These protein sources provide the necessary amino acids to preserve and increase muscle mass while limiting the amount of carbohydrates consumed. To keep their muscles strong and their energy levels consistent, seniors should make an effort to eat enough protein each day.

2. Fiber and Digestive Health:

A low-carb diet may cause you to consume less dietary fiber, which is detrimental to your digestive tract. Constipation is a common issue among seniors that can be alleviated by consuming adequate amounts of fiber. Include foods high in fiber and low in carbohydrates, such as leafy greens, seeds, and non-starchy vegetables.

Furthermore, choosing complete, unprocessed meals over refined ones while adhering to a low-carb lifestyle may result in an increase in fiber intake. Fiber assists seniors who are trying to control their portion sizes by making them feel fuller for longer periods of time, in addition to encouraging regular bowel movements.

3. Vitamins and Minerals for Seniors on a Low Carb Diet:

While a low-carb diet has numerous health benefits, it may inadvertently result in a decrease in the intake of vital vitamins and minerals. Seniors must be very mindful of the nutrients they eat to prevent deficits. Vital vitamins and minerals to consider are calcium, vitamin D, B vitamins, and potassium.

Dairy products, leafy greens, and fortified meals are rich sources of calcium and vitamin D. Low-carb vegetables and lean proteins are good sources of B vitamins; avocados and other nuts are good sources of potassium.

These sources can be incorporated into a well-rounded, low-carb diet to help seniors reduce their carbohydrate intake without sacrificing overall health.

"SENIORS, THRIVE ON LOW CARBS, NOT LIMITS!"

CHAPTER 4:

LOW CARB BREAKFAST IDEAS FOR SENIOR VITALITY

A low-carb diet can be a smart choice for seniors who wish to maintain their general well-being and vigor because our nutritional needs vary as we age. Breakfast is often regarded as the most important meal of the day since it provides us with the energy we need to begin our days. Particularly seniors should focus on nutrient-dense diets that sustain long-term energy levels without adversely influencing blood sugar levels.

The following are some hearty senior breakfast ideas that adhere to the Ultimate Low Carb Diet's recommendations:

1. Scrambled Eggs with Spinach and Feta:

Because they are a fantastic source of protein and other nutrients, eggs make an excellent breakfast option.

Scramble eggs with a handful of fresh spinach and a sprinkle of feta cheese for a high-energy, low-carb breakfast.

2. Greek Yogurt Parfait:

Greek yogurt, which is high in protein and probiotics, helps to maintain digestive health. To make a parfait, top Greek yogurt with a small quantity of low-sugar fruit and chopped almonds for flavor and texture.

3. Smoked Salmon and Avocado Wraps:

For those who enjoy a substantial breakfast, smoked salmon and avocado wraps are a fantastic choice. Place avocado slices and smoked salmon between lettuce leaves or nori seaweed, then drizzle with a little olive oil.

4. Chia Seed Pudding:

Supermeal Chia seeds are low in carbs and high in fiber. Mix them with cinnamon, unsweetened almond milk, and a small amount of vanilla essence. Put it in the refrigerator for the night and wake up to a pudding-like, nutrient-rich breakfast.

5. **Veggie Omelet:**

Incorporate tomatoes, bell peppers, and mushrooms into an omelette along with other colorful, low-carb vegetables. Add some cheese and herbs to give it additional flavor.

6. **Cottage Cheese and Berries:**

Cottage cheese is a low-carb, high-protein option. Top it with a handful of fresh, low-sugar berries, such raspberries or strawberries, for a pleasant and satisfying breakfast.

The Significance of Breakfast

Sustained Energy: Eating breakfast helps to stabilize blood sugar levels and replenish your energy after a restful night's sleep. Seniors on a low-carb diet can prevent the high-carb meal-related energy spikes and crashes by making smart dietary choices.

Cognitive performance: Eating a nutritious breakfast helps seniors remember things better and think more clearly. Diets low in carbohydrates can improve focus and reduce the risk of cognitive decline.

Start Your Metabolism: Eating a nutritious meal causes your metabolism to speed up. Diets low in carbohydrates encourage the body to use stored fat as an energy source, which is good for overall health and weight loss.

Energizing Senior Low-Carb Breakfast Ideas:

Protein-Packed Eggs: Eggs are a terrific option because they're low in carbs and high in protein. They provide you with essential nutrients and keep you feeling satisfied and full.

Greek yogurt with Berries: Choose the plain kind, which is higher in protein and probiotics. Add a handful of fresh berries to increase your intake of antioxidants and fiber without the added carbohydrates found in sweet yogurts.

Nutrient-Dense Smoothies: Blend spinach, avocado, unsweetened almond milk, and a scoop of protein powder to create low-carb smoothies that are high in healthy fats, vitamins, and minerals.

Chia Seed Pudding: Chia seeds are high in fiber and good lipids, but they also have a low-carb sweetness. Blend them with almond milk and your favorite low-carb sweetener to create a filling pudding that can be prepared ahead of time.

Vegetable Omelet: Pack your omelette full of low-carb vegetables including spinach, bell peppers, and mushrooms. This delicious alternative adds just the right amount of vitamins and minerals without packing on the carbs.

Avocado Toast: Swap out the toast for a slice of avocado. For a delicious low-carb twist on a classic favorite, top it with cherry tomatoes, smoked salmon, or a poached egg.

Recipes for a Powerful, Nutrient-Started Morning

A nutrient-dense breakfast is an essential for seniors following the ultimate low-carb diet. A balanced meal increases your metabolism and provides you with the essential nutrition and energy you need to maintain an active and healthy lifestyle. Here are some delicious low-carb recipe ideas to make sure you get your morning

1. Veggie Omelet with Avocado

Ingredients:

Two ovum

1/4 cup of bell peppers, chopped

1/4 cup of spinach, cut finely

1/4 cup of mushrooms, sliced

A quarter of an avocado, sliced

To taste, add salt and pepper.

Whisk the eggs and then pour them into a nonstick pan that has been heated. Add the diced vegetables and heat until the omelet is done. Fold it in half, then place sliced avocado on top and serve. This omelet's high protein and healthy fat content will keep you satiated throughout the morning.

2. Greek Yogurt Parfait

Ingredients:

Half a cup of Greek yogurt without sugar

1/4 cup of mixed berries, either blue, rasp, or strawberry

Half a teaspoon of finely chopped nuts (almonds, walnuts, or pecans)

If preferred, add half a teaspoon of honey.

Combine Greek yogurt, sliced almonds, and mixed berries in a glass or bowl. Drizzle with honey if preferred. This breakfast parfait supports healthy digestion and helps to keep blood sugar levels steady. It has a lot of fiber, protein, and few carbs.

3. Smoked Salmon and Cream Cheese Roll-Ups

Ingredients:

Two smoked salmon slices

A double portion of cream cheese

two or three thin cucumber slices

Decoratively add fresh dill.

Drizzle the smoked salmon chunks with cream cheese, place slices of cucumber on top, and roll up. Add a handful of fresh dill on top. These roll-ups are low in carbs and high in heart-healthy omega-3 fatty acids.

4. Pudding with Chia Seeds

Ingredients:

Two chia seed tablespoons

A half-cup of plain almond milk

1/4 teaspoon of unadulterated vanilla

1/4 cup unsweetened shredded coconut or raw berries (for topping)

Mix the almond milk, vanilla essence, and chia seeds in a jar or other container. Refrigerate for several hours or overnight to allow it to thicken. Top with fresh berries or some shredded coconut. Chia seed pudding is a high-fiber, low-carb, and high-nutrient breakfast option.

CHAPTER 5:

SATISFYING LOW CARB LUNCH AND DINNER RECIPES FOR THE ULTIMATE LOW CARB DIET FOR SENIORS

Seniors may worry that following a low-carb diet will mean giving up flavor and satisfaction. The good news is that with a little creativity and the right ingredients, you can have filling low-carb lunch and dinner options that satisfy both your taste buds and your health. In this post, we'll examine a few hearty recipes that can help you reduce your carb intake and enhance your overall health.

Suitable Lunch Ideas:

Salad with grilled chicken and avocado: **A hearty dish with fresh avocados, vibrant greens, and a tangy vinaigrette. For seniors, this salad is satisfying and nourishing because it is high in protein and healthy fats.**

Pesto-Garden Zucchini Noodles: Instead of using conventional spaghetti, use spiralized zucchini noodles. Drizzle with homemade pesto sauce made with basil. This recipe packs a nutrient- and flavor-packed punch while using less carbs.

Broccoli and Cauliflower Soup: This hearty and creamy soup is made with broccoli, cauliflower, and a small amount of cheese. This soup is great for keeping warm on a cold day because it has a high fiber level and low carbohydrate load.

Appetizing Dinners to Control Carbs:

Baked Salmon with Garlic Butter: A simple yet tasty recipe that consists of salmon fillets seasoned with garlic butter and roasted vegetables. After having lean protein and healthy fats, you will feel energized and satisfied.

Stuffed Chicken Breast with Mushrooms and Spinach: A delicious chicken breast stuffed with sautéed mushrooms and spinach is called a stuffed chicken breast. This is a low-carb culinary creation that is sure to impress.

Pizza with a Cauliflower Crust: Enjoy the flavors of classic pizza without the added carbohydrates. A cauliflower crust topped with your favorite low-carb toppings will offer a guilt-free supper option that seniors will enjoy.

These meals are tasty and thoughtful of senior citizens' dietary needs. Meals reduced in carbohydrates can reduce the risk of acquiring chronic illnesses, assist control weight, and maintain stable blood sugar levels.

The key is to prioritize eating lots of fresh produce, lean meats, healthy fats, and greens. By including these satisfying low-carb lunch and dinner ideas into your regular meal, you may begin the finest low-carb diet for seniors and enjoy every mouthful. a healthy appetite

"IN THE BOOK OF LIFE, SENIORS WRITE THEIR CHAPTER WITH LOW CARB WISDOM."

CHAPTER 6:

SNACKS AND DESSERTS: LOW CARB INDULGENCES

Eating low-carbohydrate cuisine as a senior means enjoying life's small pleasures in addition to remaining nourished. Your major meals should be the foundation of your nutritional journey when following the "Ultimate Low Carb Diet for Seniors," but it's also critical to address your cravings for snacks and sweets during the times in between meals. In this section, we'll examine ways to satisfy your cravings without consuming too many carbohydrates.

Healthy Low-Carb Treats

Snacking in moderation is essential to a successful low-carb diet, particularly for older persons. It helps prevent overindulging during meals and maintains steady energy levels. Here, we offer you a selection of healthful, low-carb snack options that are not only delicious but also nourishing.

From a dish of almonds to crispy vegetable sticks with a delectable dip, we have everything you need. These foods can help keep your blood sugar levels constant and your energy levels high since they contain healthy fats, fiber, and protein. Seniors who want to maintain their energy and appropriately manage their weight should choose healthy, low-carb snacks.

Desserts for Seniors' Sweet Taste Cravings Without Feeling Shameful

Sweet tooth cravings are common, but they don't have to prevent you from achieving your low-carb goals. We understand that older adults may have a preference for traditional sweets and will never tire of flavor.

You may find a range of guilt-free dessert options in this section that will entice your taste senses without going overboard with the quantity you consume.

These desserts are designed to have the most flavor and the fewest carbohydrates possible. Examples of such desserts are rich berry parfaits, creamy avocado chocolate mousse, and warm apple compote with spices and cinnamon.

If you employ inventive ingredient substitutions and sensible portion control, you may indulge in these delicious treats without feeling guilty or compromising your nutritional goals.

Remember that the "Ultimate Low Carb Diet for Seniors" is all about moderation and creativity. Snacks and desserts can enhance rather than detract from your low-carb journey. They can be a tasty complement. Enjoy the flavors, accept the reduced-carb options, and look after your physical and mental well-being.

CHAPTER 7:

DINING OUT AND SPECIAL OCCASIONS

Navigating Low Carb Choices at Restaurants

Dining out and celebrating are often times of joy and excess, but they can also provide challenges for people following low-carb diets, such as the Ultimate Low Carb Diet for Seniors. You may enjoy these wonderful moments and maintain your diet plan at the same time by making smart choices and employing a few strategic tactics.

1. Make a Plan: Before you attend a restaurant or special event, take some time to familiarize yourself with the menu options. Many restaurants now include nutritional information on their websites, allowing you to make advance selections among low-carb meals. Knowing what to order ahead of time can help you stay focused.

2. Accept Protein: Lean proteins like steak, fish, and grilled chicken are commonly offered on restaurant menus. These high-protein options are excellent for low-carb diets and

pair nicely with non-starchy vegetables or salads. You are welcome to change your order to accommodate your dietary requirements and preferences.

3. Avoid Hidden Carbs: Unidentified carbs can be found in sauces, dressings, and condiments. Use simple, low-carb dressings for salads, such as vinegar and olive oil. Ask for the sauce on the side so you can be sure you use the appropriate quantity.

4. Swap Sides: In lieu of high-carb sides like rice or potatoes, many restaurants allow you to request low-carb sides like steamed vegetables or a side salad. Make one simple substitution and your carbohydrate intake can change considerably.

5. Adopt Portion Control: The size of restaurant meals is a regular issue. Consider sharing a dish with a dining companion at the beginning of the meal or asking for a to-go box so you may bag half for later. You may maintain your carbohydrate intake and prevent overindulgence by doing this.

Taking Pleasure in Low-Carb Eating During Holidays:

Special occasions and festivities sometimes include festive lunches and get-togethers. Even though sticking to a low-carb diet during these times might seem challenging, it is completely achievable with some deliberate choices and an optimistic outlook.

1. Bring a dish: Consider bringing a dish that you enjoy that is low in carbohydrates if you're attending a potluck or an event where you get to pick the menu. This ensures that there will be a minimum of one option that meets your nutritional goals.

2. Communicate Your Preferences: Don't be afraid to inform the host or staff members of the foods you are allergic to. Many hosts are accommodating and willing to change meals or accommodate your dietary needs. Never be afraid to ask for adjustments to your order when dining out.

3. Make Protein and Veggies a Priority: Pay particular attention to lean proteins and non-starchy vegetables during celebration meals. These meals are often part of the traditional celebratory buffet and can be consumed guilt-free.

4. Mindful Indulgence: While maintaining a low-carb diet is crucial, there are occasions when you deserve to reward yourself. If you do want to indulge, do it mindfully and slowly before guilt-free returning to your low-carb diet.

With these tips, you may follow the Ultimate Low Carb Diet for Seniors and still manage special occasions like eating out. Remember that eating may still be enjoyable and rewarding in social settings and can also improve your overall health and well-being.

CHAPTER 8:

LONG-TERM SUCCESS AND SUSTAINABLE LOW CARB LIVING

Seniors who embark on a low-carb journey towards improved health have hope for long-term success and sustainable well-being ahead of them. Adopting a low-carb lifestyle means putting long-term health and vibrancy ahead of short-term remedies.

This article explores the key elements of adhering to a low-carb lifestyle and ensuring long-term senior heath through a low-carb diet, all within the context of the "Ultimate Low Carb Diet for Seniors."

Maintaining My Low-Carb Lifestyle

Maintaining a low-carb lifestyle requires commitment, just like any other long-term achievement. Remembering that this is a long-term shift rather than a short-term fix is crucial. To stay faithful:

Education: Continue to learn about the benefits of maintaining a low-carb lifestyle. Your commitment may be strengthened when you realize the advantages for your health.

Meal Planning: Make the effort to cook enticing, low-carb meals. When you enjoy something more, it's simpler to stick to a diet.

Accountability: Discuss your experience with friends and family. A strong support system could inspire you and help you stay on track.

Variety: Examine a wide range of low-carb recipes and ingredients. By mixing things up, you can keep your commitment from getting boring.

Adaptation: As you age, your nutritional needs may change. Be flexible and prepared to modify your low-carb approach as needed.

A Low-Carbohydrate Diet for Healthy Aging Throughout Life

The "Ultimate Low Carb Diet for Seniors" has the potential to enhance your life in many ways. By adopting this low-carb lifestyle, you are investing in your long-term health and well-being. A few benefits are as follows:

Weight control: By maintaining a healthy weight, seniors on low-carb diets are less likely to experience health issues associated with obesity.

Steady Blood Sugar: People who already have diabetes or who are at risk for the condition can keep their blood sugar levels steady by following a low-carb diet.

Improved Heart Health: A diet reduced in carbohydrates can help reduce the risk of heart disease, improve cholesterol profiles, and lower blood pressure.

Better Brain Health: Because carbs have a direct impact on cognitive function, a low-carb diet can help you preserve the health of your brain as you age.

Energy and Vitality: Elderly people who eat a low-carb diet frequently talk about feeling more alive and full of energy.

CONCLUSION

In summary, adopting an ultra-low-carb diet for seniors provides a comprehensive approach to nutrition that is in line with both the health requirements of the aging population and a dedication to environmental sustainability.

It is critical for dietitians to understand the special dietary needs of seniors, including the need of maintaining a balance between macronutrients, especially in light of their decreased physical activity levels and potential aging-related metabolic alterations.

Seniors on a low-carb diet should choose foods that are high in nutrients and sustainable for the environment, as well as high in vital vitamins and minerals. Promoting the use of seasonal produce that is acquired locally helps regional agriculture and lessens the carbon footprint that comes with long-distance driving.

Furthermore, by minimizing the ecological impact of animal agriculture, placing an emphasis on plant-based protein sources like legumes and nuts is consistent with an environmentally sustainable diet and improves cardiovascular health.

Moreover, a low-carb diet for seniors that incorporates whole, minimally processed foods promotes a holistic approach to health. This reduces the environmental impact of producing and discarding highly processed meals in addition to meeting dietary needs. In order to support the preservation of marine ecosystems, it is imperative to emphasize the significance of sustainable fishing methods while advocating seafood as a source of protein.

A dietitian should place a high priority on educating clients about mindful consumption, waste reduction, and the environmental effects of food choices when promoting an optimal low-carb diet for seniors.

Seniors can optimize their own well-being with a low-carb diet that is both ecologically conscientious and nutritionally balanced, while also contributing to a more sustainable future by raising awareness of the connection between eating habits and the health of the world.

In the end, encouraging sustainable eating habits is crucial for maintaining the planet's health for future generations in addition to being beneficial to individual health.

HAPPY COOKING

www.ingramcontent.com/pod-product-compliance
Lightning Source LLC
Chambersburg PA
CBHW070740260726
48660CB00007B/2914